# How to Stay Young

*Science-Based Guide for Enhancing Health as You Age.*

Dr. Stella Reynolds

# TABLE OF CONTENTS

# Introduction

The keys to long life and good health may be found in the domains of disciplined living, wise decision-making, and in-depth knowledge of the human body, not in far-off regions or mythical seas.

These precise strategies are what "How to Stay Young: Science-Based Guide for Enhancing Health as You Age" aims to reveal. This book isn't about making improbable claims or breaking the laws of nature. Understanding our body's wonderful mechanisms and knowing how to maintain their functioning at their best as the years pass are key components of this.

Growing older is about more than just the passage of time; it's also about the effects of the choices we've made along the way.

This book is designed to help you gain the knowledge and abilities required to navigate your golden years with grace, vigor, and a revitalized sense of purpose.

Keep yourself fresh in body, intellect, and soul, as well as in heart. Within, you will find the science of aging gracefully.

# Chapter 1

## Get Younger From The Inside Out

Whether we like to admit it or not, most people over the age of 25 are interested in staying young. And you've undoubtedly thought about doing a little differently than your grandparents did if you've seen what a lifetime of hard living looked like on them. Although your lifestyle has a huge impact on how your genes manifest themselves in the body, genetics do play a considerable part in how well or poorly you age.

Positive lifestyle modifications can significantly reduce the risk of chronic illnesses including heart disease, diabetes, Alzheimer's, and even cancer. Step away from the Botox needle and toward these very effective youth-preserving remedies instead if you want to lengthen your "healthspan"—the number of healthy years you may enjoy:

**1)      Concentrate      On      The      Edible Youth-Maintainers.**

What you eat is at the top of the list of actions that either prolong life or drain it. True medicine comes from nature—appropriate meals.  If you want to feel and look good for as long as possible, opt for fresh, organic, or farmer's market vegetables and meats. They'll fill up your tank with antioxidants, polyphenols, and countless other nutrients that are beneficial to your overall health.

Think vitality, vibrancy, glowing skin, healthy hair, etc. Big Macs, bangers, and beer will not suffice as a diet. to increase the frequency of eating organic, healthy food without going bankrupt.

## 2) Get Rid Of The #1 Youth-Drainer.

What occupies the top position in the youth-sucking food chain? It is sugar. Remove it as well as agave and honey. The deadly sweet thing kills slowly, sneakily, and addictively while compromising the immune system and promoting the feared "diseases of aging." In essence, sugar rots you from the inside out by destroying cell membranes and forming deposits on your organs that look like rust. Have wrinkling? On your skin, the greatest organ in your body, you can see the 'rust' caused by sugar.

What is the simplest strategy to handle sugar's disadvantages? Starting with the obvious sources, such as cereal, cookies, candies, soda, and fruit juice, stop using them. Have a sweet tooth? Then, to assist in decreasing the absorption of sugar and reducing blood sugar spikes and crashes, munch on a small serving of low-sugar berries.

If you wish, sprinkle the berries with a pinch of cinnamon and a little flax or chia seeds.

## 3) Avoid Meals That Are Hard On Your Body.

Fast food is, of course, included in the group of processed foods that come in a close second for accelerating aging. For a few reasons, they're bad for your body. To begin with, almost all processed meals include a significant amount of artificial substances, the long-term consequences of which are either extremely dubious, significantly harmful to your health, or even cancerous.

There are a lot of chemical additives, including artificial colors, fake flavors, fillers, vegetable oils, preservatives, and salt. We don't yet fully understand the damage they may do over time, which is even more alarming, but I can assure you that vigorous health won't be one of the results.

We are aware of the connection between eating processed foods and a higher risk of obesity, diabetes, cancer, and heart disease. entire, unprocessed foods? Everything is fantastic. There is no need to be concerned about cheap, pesticide-filled, factory-farmed, genetically engineered ingredients. There are no secret sugars (such as disaccharides, galactose, hexanol, inversol, pentose, sucanat, etc.) that only a food scientist would be able to identify. No drawbacks, no issues.

## 4) Accept The Crucial Anti-Aging Activity That Involves Your Pillow.

Sleeping is never a waste of time. A key component of the anti-aging equation and a necessity for staying young is deep, peaceful, restorative sleep, especially REM sleep when dreams occur. A lot of the symptoms that people associate with aging, such as aches, pains, and low energy, are the body's way of informing you that it needs more (and better) sleep.

Even though it might not appear like anything is occurring when you go to bed, your body is recovering during that time. Sleep encourages autophagy, the cellular recycling process carried out overnight by your glymphatic system, which maintains all of your cells, muscles, and organs. The body separates the salvageable components and recycles them to utilize them for energy and to generate new cells rather than discarding the sick or inferior cells. Nice, huh?

So, the glymphatic system is unable to function when you have a propensity for under-sleeping. There isn't time to "take out the trash." As cellular waste accumulates in the brain, you become disoriented and groggy.

By allowing your body the downtime it requires to conduct its cleansing, you may help prevent neurological illness and decline.

**5) Don't Merely Stand (or Sit) Still.**

The fastest route to premature aging is inactivity, so get moving right away and don't stop! Fitness has somewhat slipped to the sidelines over the last two epidemic years. It's time to start moving around again. You don't have to sign up for boot camp tomorrow (unless that's your thing), but you should get back into the habit of moving regularly and frequently. It's about moving as much as you can during your normal daily activities rather than scheduling a single gym visit to fit in between a day at the office and an evening on the sofa.

Take every opportunity to be active. Beyond the age of 40, it's OK for exercise to focus more on movement, motion, and mobility and less on severe exertion and pushing your body to its physical limits. The secret to physically aging well is avoiding damage (as in, if it hurts, don't do it), keeping the joints lubricated, and keeping the muscles supple and ready to fire.

Physical activity prevents stress and depression, boosts circulation, encourages better sleep, strengthens the immune system, lowers the risk of chronic illnesses, and keeps the body and mind healthy and alert. So, after dinner, how about a stroll?

**6) Slow Down The Aging Process Every Day.**

Slowing down the aging process requires periodic time-outs for your mind and body. While a week spent by the sea isn't always possible, a calming getaway in the form of a meditation practice can be.

Spending time in meditation reduces blood pressure and slows brain aging. Additionally, it lengthens your telomeres, which are the caps that preserve your DNA strands and have a significant impact on how well you age (the longer they are, the younger you will be).

All you need is a quiet place and 10 to 20 minutes a day to get the rewards of meditation, which include benefits for greater focus, mood, and sleep. If you're not a "sitter," what should you do? Then, start a tranquil practice that fits you: knitting, coloring, wandering in the woods, or whatever quiet, relaxing activity you love doing unplugged and without interruption.

**7) Get Rid Of The Toxins That Age You.**

It never hurts to consider eliminating toxins from your life, whether they are chemical, physical, or emotional, when it comes to slowing down the aging process. I strongly advise you to stop smoking if you're still doing it or even if you only occasionally slip one in. Any quantity of smoking increases the chance of heart disease, lung cancer, cataracts, and a long list of other serious illnesses. Just refuse.

The same is true for drinking; it is not beneficial to you. A glass of wine once or twice a week to go with a special meal is OK, but any more than that puts you at risk for health problems due to overconsumption. Alcohol may cause your gray matter to shrink, which will negatively impact your brain function over time. Your organs will also suffer, as will your face (the substance is bad for your complexion).

You don't need another quick ager, do you? the unhealthy connections and harmful individuals in your life. Finding a gradual approach to phase those "toxins" out, if at all feasible, is a crucial step to take to protect your health now and in the future because of the stress they contribute to your life.

**8) Age Less With A Strong Case Of The Giggles.**

I also strongly advise having a bout of the giggles at least once every day as another anti-aging practice. Laughter strengthens the immune system by enhancing the activity of T cells, or "killer cells," which assist our bodies in battling cancer and infections. No matter where you are on the aging path, it also helps lower blood pressure and cortisol levels, relieves discomfort, and can also help balance blood sugar.

# Chapter 2

## Skincare and Aging Gracefully

As we embrace this natural process of aging, our skin changes as well. Aging gracefully is a lovely journey that comes with time. While we cannot stop the passage of time, we may take proactive measures to age gracefully and keep our skin looking healthy and young. In this blog, we'll dig into a wealth of anti-aging skincare procedures and recommendations to give you the information you need to accept age with assurance and brightness.

**The Foundation: Basics of Skincare**

With a solid foundation in skincare fundamentals, start your road toward aging gracefully. Develop a regular regimen that includes cleaning, toning, moisturizing, and protecting your skin from UV radiation. These essential actions establish the foundation for a youthful, healthy complexion that fights aging.

## Protect Your Skin: Wearing Sunscreen is a Must-Have!

Protection from the elements, especially the sun, is the foundation of anti-aging skincare. One of the main reasons for early aging is sun damage. In any condition, make sunscreen your constant ally. Use sunscreen to shield your skin from UVA and UVB rays. Search for a broad-spectrum lotion with an SPF of at least 30.

## Inside and Outside hydration

By putting moisture first, you may increase the natural resilience of your skin. To nourish your skin from the inside out, drink plenty of water. Hyaluronic acid-enriched skincare products should be used in conjunction with this internal hydration. This miraculous substance has the amazing capacity to hold moisture, giving your skin a dewy, fresh appearance.

## Excellent Moisturization

Achieve a soft, radiant complexion by moisturizing carefully. Choose a luxurious, moisturizing moisturizer that is suitable for your skin type. In addition to feeling smoother, a well-moisturized complexion reduces the appearance of fine wrinkles, a sign of aging skin.

## Influence of Retinoids

Utilize the anti-aging properties of retinoids, which are vitamin A derivatives, to successfully fight the effects of aging. Retinoids increase the production of collagen, speed up cell renewal, and significantly lessen wrinkle visibility. To find the finest products for your skin's requirements, get advice from a dermatologist and gradually introduce retinoids into your regimen.

## Antioxidant Allies

Antioxidants like vitamin C can strengthen the defenses of your skin. These helpful buddies combat the free radicals that hasten premature aging. As part of your skincare routine, seamlessly include antioxidant-rich serums or creams to protect your skin from environmental aggressors.

## Gentle Exfoliation

Use the advantages of routine exfoliation to remove dead, dull skin cells and reveal a revitalized appearance. Give mild exfoliants that respect the equilibrium of your skin's priority. To preserve skin clarity without overburdening your complexion, aim for exfoliating sessions once to twice a week.

## Beauty Sleep: A Friend for Your Skin

Make getting enough sleep a priority since it is a haven for rest and healing for your skin. Aiming for 7-9 hours of quality sleep each night can guarantee that you awaken with a refreshed and beautiful complexion, which is proof of the effectiveness of beauty sleep in defying aging.

## Inside-Out Nourishment

By adopting a diet that is well-balanced and full of fruits, vegetables, lean proteins, and healthy fats, you can promote skin health from the inside out. Omega-3 fatty acids provide your skin with essential nutrition for its journey through time and are found in foods like salmon and flaxseed.

**Management of Stress and Self-Care**

Chronic stress can hasten aging and deplete the vitality of your skin. Use stress-relieving methods to combat this, such as yoga, meditation, or spending time in nature. Set aside time for self-care to look after your skin and general wellbeing.

Let us keep in mind that aging gracefully is a comprehensive endeavor that integrates inner and exterior care as we welcome the unstoppable march of time. You can celebrate the knowledge that comes with each new day by adopting these anti-aging skincare treatments and tricks. Your skin, a canvas that records your journey, ought to be treated with respect for the life it has already experienced. By taking care of your skin, you honor the tale it conveys, one that exudes assurance, brilliance, and the grace that only time can provide.

# Chapter 3

## The Power of Proactive Health Choices

The significance of well-being in life's journey is akin to a guiding light illuminating the way to fruitful living. This chapter examines a way of thinking that appeals to people looking to take a proactive approach to their health journey. Explore the foundations and possible advantages of putting preventative healthcare first.

This tale encourages readers to manage their well-being with an empowered viewpoint, connecting with the core principles of preventative healthcare, via accessible expressions and incisive analyses.

## The Vitality of Proactivity

A person's readiness to address health issues before they get worse is referred to as proactivity about health. This method includes making educated decisions, taking preventative action, and cultivating a lifestyle that is supportive of total well-being as opposed to only responding to health difficulties.

## Making Lifestyle Choices

Conscious lifestyle choices are one of the pillars of proactive health strategy. These decisions—from nutrition to exercise, sleep to stress reduction—lay the groundwork for a strong sense of well-being. Taking control of our diets, exercising, and embracing mindfulness are pieces of the proactive health jigsaw that fit together seamlessly.

## Setting Preventive Measures as a Priority

The cornerstone of proactive health is prevention, which is frequently hailed as the best medication.

The proactive arsenal against possible health threats includes routine checkups, vaccines, and health screenings. By identifying problems early, people may take action before things get worse, according to the overriding idea of proactive well-being.

## Empowerment via Knowledge

An empowered person is well-informed. People who are aware of health issues, symptoms, and risk factors are better equipped to see warning signals. By encouraging proactive decision-making, this empowerment enables prompt treatments and lessens the potential effects of health issues.

## The Function of Mental Health

Proactivity encompasses mental and physical health. Mental resilience is increased through acknowledging feelings, getting support, and using stress-reduction tactics. A proactive approach to mental health recognizes the link between the mind and body and promotes holistic wellness.

**Establishing Consistency**

The core of a proactive health journey is consistency. Whether it's sticking to a workout schedule, eating a balanced diet, or regularly practicing relaxation methods, the cumulative effect of tiny, deliberate activities over time multiplies well-being.

Work in Partnership with Healthcare Professionals

A proactive strategy cannot exist by itself. Collaboration with medical experts is crucial because it enables people to create tailored health programs. To ensure that activities are in line with individual needs, routine consultations, health advice, and monitoring all contribute to proactive management.

## The Value of Early Detection

Early detection is a key component of a proactive approach to health. The goal of preventive healthcare is to identify possible health problems in the early stages by encouraging people to get routine tests and checkups. People can take prompt action to treat and lessen the effects of illnesses like high blood pressure, diabetes, or cancer through early detection. Early identification perfectly complements the tenets of preventive healthcare since it improves treatment results and lessens the need for drastic measures.

## Education for Individual Empowerment

The foundation of preventative healthcare is education. People may make wise decisions about their health when they are equipped with knowledge about healthy lifestyles, risk factors, and preventative actions. Resources and educational initiatives offer important insights into the advantages of keeping a healthy weight, being physically active, and controlling stress. Preventive healthcare promotes proactive decisions that can enhance health outcomes and a greater quality of life by empowering people with the correct information.

**Being Healthy Requires Daily Practice.**

We're all considering protection, whether your children are putting on backpacks for a new school year or you have returned to the office. Masks and reducing our risk of exposure are hot topics right now, and we're flooded with news articles and social media messages about them.

However, we don't talk enough about the daily lifestyle decisions that we make. Proactive self-care is the foundation of well-being. These are the preventive steps we may take to enhance our general health and, consequently, our prognoses if we contract a cold, the flu, or SARS-CoV-2.

Our condition of health and wellness is the result of the accumulation of all of our daily routines, thoughts, and deeds. As Benjamin Franklin once remarked, "An ounce of prevention is worth a pound of cure." Our routine activities could either make our health worse or better. By making investments in your health, you significantly lower your risk of getting sick, and if you do, you improve your chances of recovering quickly.

***Five Ways to Maintain a Strong Immune System***

**1. Get Sufficient Sleep**

The adage "An apple a day keeps the doctor away" is almost as well-known as "You should get 8 hours of sleep every night." However, is it true? Recent studies on circadian rhythms support a different opinion. Stop focusing on the 8-hour threshold and start considering what appears to work best for you if you've been attempting to change a sleep pattern that doesn't meet it.

The reality is that everyone's sleep patterns are different. Although less than 7 has been demonstrated to enhance the chance of unfavorable health occurrences, the average amount of sleep recommended is 8, yet you may discover that you function just as well with 7. Perhaps your spouse or adolescent requires nine to operate, plus a bit more if the body is healing from a sickness or injury. Make sure you're receiving what you need by finding what works.

Try to set a regular wake-up time and attempt to get to bed on time. The key is routine and consistency.

## 2. Get Adequate Rest

You may be thinking, "Isn't that what I do while I sleep?" Yes and no, I suppose. While there are seven different forms of rest, sleep is only one of them.

*Physical: savasana, catnaps, and sleep*

*Mental: Taking frequent pauses from work*

*Take a break from devices, close your eyes, and unplug for sensory purposes.*

*Get creative by spending time in nature or visiting a museum.*

*Emotionally, communicate honestly and let go of the need to appease others.*

*Socializing: Try to engage in deeper conversations rather than small-talk at social gatherings rather than forcing oneself to go.*

*Spirituality: meaningful connections with others, meditation*

Include scheduled, actual downtime in your everyday activities. Rest is crucial for both our physical and emotional well-being, and these fulfilling methods to unwind support our relationships with one another, our surroundings, and our loved ones.

## 3. Give Your Body Healthy Food.

The foundation of good health is a healthy diet. There are several fad diets out there that make different, sometimes conflicting claims regarding things like fat consumption, fasting, the proper quantity of meat and dairy, anti-inflammatory foods, and much more. Investigating the scientific justifications for these diets might lead you down a disorienting rabbit hole. Nobody has time for that. If you're not a dietician, you probably have more important things to accomplish.

Eating genuine, unprocessed food—fruits, vegetables, and meats—and consuming more fruits and vegetables than meat is the most crucial part of nutrition.

## 4. Stay Hydrated Regularly.

It's common to grab a large glass of iced water after a vigorous workout or in the sweltering heat of the day. We act without contemplating it. What about when you get up in the morning or are on your way to work? How about drinking a glass of water before supper or choosing water for a sugary snack in the middle of the day?

You probably don't carry a water bottle with you unless you live in a dry area that continually makes you thirsty. Yet you ought to be. Maintaining proper hydration is crucial for our bodies to flush out waste, regulate our internal temperature, lubricate our joints, and preserve delicate tissues. You stay awake if you stay hydrated!

## 5. Stress Management

The same principle applies to what's going on in our thoughts in the same way that we are what we consume. Our bodies and minds suffer when we are under stress. Stress consumes us continually, and it manifests.

"The most pernicious underlying cause of illness is chronic stress. Both the emotional aspect of stress—"I feel overwhelmed"—and the physical aspect of stress—"increased heart rate, blood pressure, blood sugars, brain fog, increased central body fat, etc.—are brought on by chemicals like cortisol and adrenaline. Techniques for reducing stress and managing it are essential for achieving good health.

The growth mindset and mindfulness both aim to control how the body reacts to stress on both physical and mental levels. William James once observed, "Our capacity to select one idea over another is the best defense against stress.

Meditating in the morning is one strategy to combat stress proactively. Regular mindful meditation practice has been demonstrated in studies to assist people in managing stress, anxiety, and discomfort. It also falls under one of the previously listed five categories of rest, providing a double dose of health for both your body and mind.

*Conclusion*

The empowerment narrative reverberates with the proactive well-being story. By adopting a proactive attitude, people create a story of energy, resilience, and deliberate living. This journey is a celebration of taking control, making decisions that are in line with well-being, and developing routines that honor the gift of health.

The embrace of empowerment is the compass directing people toward a life that embraces health as a treasured possession, representing the essence of proactive healthcare, as the path toward proactive well-being progresses.

# Chapter 4

## Optimizing  Brain-Gut Health

The gut-brain axis refers to the intricate and complex relationship between your stomach and brain. To keep your mind and body functioning efficiently and harmoniously, signals must travel in both directions, from your brain down to your gut and vice versa.

Your gut health directly affects your mood, and vice versa. More connections between the stomach and brain than previously believed are being discovered through new research on the gut-brain axis. These discoveries have the amazing potential to aid those with digestive problems by enhancing brain health. Similarly, those with brain or mood disorders may benefit from improving their gut health.

## How Gut Health Is Affected by Stress and Emotions

You've likely felt your gut-brain axis in action if you've ever experienced butterflies in the stomach before a big test or presentation. Your digestion slows down when you're under a lot of stress so that your muscles can fight or run. Whether your worry is caused by an actual threat or just an imagined one, the same bodily response manifests.

Your body responds in the same manner via the gut-brain axis whether you're in a life-threatening crisis or are extremely stressed out about an impending deadline. Pain, nausea, and other associated problems may be brought on by this disturbance of your digestive system.

It is simple to see how stress and other emotions may have an impact on the stomach given the tight connections between the gut and brain. Your digestive tract and stomach are frequently where you sense emotions like fear, sorrow, rage, or feeling nervous or depressed. You may feel discomfort and bloating when these feelings drive your digestive processes to speed up or slow down excessively. This is why a variety of gut conditions, including Crohn's disease, colitis, irritable bowel syndrome (IBS), gastroesophageal reflux disease (GERD), or food allergies or sensitivities, can be caused by or made worse by stress and intense emotions.

## Unresolved Gut-Brain Problems: A Vicious Cycle

If left untreated, gastrointestinal problems brought on by persistent stress can send signals to your brain that trigger an increased stress response and negatively impact your mood. The final effect is a never-ending cycle of increased stress and digestive problems.

Long-term stress can also make it possible for bacteria to get through the stomach lining and into the bloodstream, activating your immune system. Chronic stress can alter your microbiome and cause gut inflammation. The gut's inflammation and microbiota can have a significant impact on many other sections of the body, not only the brain and mood, according to recent studies. They are linked to heart disease and depression as well.

## How to Eat and Relax to Improve Gut and Brain Health

Your physical and emotional health can be significantly impacted by what you eat. This is especially true when it comes to the bacteria that make up your gut microbiome. Your gut health improves when you consume more plant-based foods and foods high in fiber. That's because this kind of diet gives your beneficial gut flora their preferred meals, allowing them to develop and flourish and, in turn, assisting you in flourishing.

Foods that include prebiotics and probiotics are very effective at fostering a balanced gut flora. Prebiotics are fiber-rich foods like beans, Jerusalem artichokes, and berries that feed your gut's beneficial bacteria. Red meat and sugar intake restrictions can also be beneficial. These can help maintain a varied population of various microbial species to improve your health, which can result in a better microbiome. Additionally, they can lessen intestinal inflammation and minimize the chance of developing heart disease and depression.

**Eat More for Improved Gut and Mental/Brain Health:**

*Veggies and fruits*
*seeds and nuts*

*whole grains*

*Greek Sauerkraut*

*Eat less as well*

**Foods containing high fructose corn syrup and sugar**

*Processed Foods*

*Rough Meat*

*Relax and digest*

Research shows that people who have gastrointestinal difficulties may benefit from psychotherapy or other stress-reduction approaches. They can improve the parasympathetic "rest and digest" response, lessen inflammation, and lower the sympathetic "fight or flight" response.

**I suggest the following methods for reducing stress:**

*Guided meditation*
*Deep inhalation*
*Mindfulness*
*Restorative Yoga*

Your gut, brain, and mood will be grateful.

Your body is an intricate network of systems that communicate with one another on a variety of levels. One outstanding example is the gut-brain axis. According to research, what you eat helps your brain and mental health, in addition to your stomach and general health. Additionally, it has been demonstrated that combining a gut-healthy diet with stress-reduction methods lowers digestive discomfort and sickness.

# Chapter 5

## Longevity Foods

Some meals can give you more energy, lower your chance of becoming sick, and help you keep a healthy weight. The most nutrient-dense foods on earth must be used to feed your body if you want to live longer and be healthy. Your health and vigor will be restored when you prioritize natural plant foods in your diet, and you'll start to wonder why everyone else isn't doing the same. Spread the word and assist.

### 1. Cruciferous Vegetable

Vegetable superfoods have the rare capacity to alter human hormones, stimulate the body's natural cleansing process, and stop the development of malignant cells. To release their strong anti-cancer qualities, cruciferous vegetables should be fully chewed or consumed shredded, diced, juiced, or mixed.

Additionally, it has been shown that the cruciferous phytochemical sulforaphane shields the blood vessel wall from inflammatory signals that can cause heart disease. The foods that are highest in nutrients are cruciferous vegetables. Consume a variety of foods every day, both raw and cooked. Try cabbage, kale, Brussels sprouts, broccoli, or cauliflower.

## 2. Salad Greens

Raw cruciferous and other leafy green vegetables have less than 100 calories per pound, making them an excellent diet for weight management. Increased consumption of salads, leafy greens, or raw vegetables is linked to a lower risk of heart attack, stroke, diabetes, and several malignancies, in addition to helping people maintain a healthy weight.

Leafy greens are a good source of the carotenoids lutein and zeaxanthin, which protect the eyes from damaging light, in addition to the essential B vitamin folate. Try lettuce, kale, collard greens, mustard greens, or spinach. Carotenoids in particular, which are fat-soluble compounds present in leafy greens, have anti-inflammatory and antioxidant properties.

## 3. Nuts

Nuts are an essential part of an anti-diabetes diet because they are a high-nutrient source of good fats, plant protein, fiber, antioxidants, phytosterols, and minerals. They are also a low-glycemic item that helps lower the glycemic load of an entire meal.

Consuming nuts is linked to decreased body weight despite their high-calorie content, possibly as a result of the heart-healthy components' ability to suppress hunger. Regular nut consumption is associated with lower cholesterol levels and a lower risk of heart disease. Add chopped walnuts or sliced almonds to the top of your next salad, or include some raw cashews in a creamy salad dressing.

## 4. Seeds

Although seeds include more protein and trace elements than nuts, their nutritional profile is remarkably comparable to that of nuts in that both contain beneficial fats, minerals, and antioxidants. Omega-3 fatty acids are prevalent in flax, chia, and hemp seeds. Additionally, they are high in lignans and breast cancer-preventing phytoestrogens, including flax, chia, and sesame seeds. Pumpkin seeds are particularly high in zinc, whereas sesame seeds are high in calcium and vitamin E. Nuts and seeds should be consumed raw or very gently roasted for the greatest nutritional value. To your morning smoothie or oatmeal, try adding flax or chia seeds.

## 5. Berries

These fruits are a great source of heart-healthy antioxidants. Studies showed reductions in blood pressure, oxidative stress indicators, and total and LDL cholesterol in those who consumed blueberries or strawberries regularly for several weeks.

Berries are also beneficial for the brain and have anti-cancer characteristics; there is evidence that eating berries may help delay cognitive loss as people age. Choose tried-and-true fruits like strawberries or blueberries instead, or try something novel like goji berries.

## 6. pomegranates

A unique fruit, pomegranates contain small, crisp, juicy arils with a delectable combination of sweet and tart flavors.. More than half of the antioxidant activity of pomegranate juice is attributed to punicalagin, the most prevalent and distinctive phytochemical of the pomegranate.

The polyphenols in pomegranates have several anti-cancer, cardioprotective, and brain-healthy effects.

In different studies on senior citizens, those who drank pomegranate juice every day for 28 days outperformed those who drank a placebo drink on a memory test. To remove the fruit's edible arils, slice it around, a half-inch deep on the circumference, twist it to separate it into two pieces, and then pound the back of each piece with the back of a big spoon.

## 7. Beans

Consuming beans and other legumes regularly can help control your blood sugar, curb your appetite, and prevent colon cancer. Beans are the most nutrient-dense form of starch, and because of their slow digestion, which reduces blood sugar spikes after meals and encourages satiety, they are also an effective weight-loss and anti-diabetes diet. Colon cancer risk has been proven to be reduced by eating beans, peas, or lentils twice a week. Consuming legumes significantly reduces the risk of developing other malignancies as well. Try them all and pick your favorites. Red beans, black beans, chickpeas, lentils, and split peas are all delicious.

## 8. Mushrooms

Breast cancer risk is believed to be reduced by regular mushroom consumption.

White and Portobello Mushrooms are particularly protective against breast cancer because they contain aromatase inhibitors, which are substances that prevent the synthesis of estrogen. Numerous studies on various types of mushrooms have revealed anti-inflammatory benefits, increased immune cell activity, avoidance of DNA damage, reduced cancer cell proliferation, and suppression of angiogenesis. It is recommended to always cook mushrooms since cooking greatly reduces the amount of the potentially cancer-causing compound agaritine that is present in raw mushrooms. Regularly consume white common mushrooms, and experiment with more uncommon kinds like shiitake, oyster, maitake, or reishi.

## 9. Garlic and onions

Onions, a member of the Allium family of vegetables, have positive effects on the cardiovascular and immunological systems in addition to being anti-diabetic and anti-cancer. Prostate and stomach cancer risk are inversely correlated with an allium vegetable diet. These vegetables are prized for their organosulfur compounds, which aid in cancer prevention by detoxifying carcinogens, slowing the proliferation of cancer cells, and obstructing angiogenesis. When these substances are chewed, crushed, or chopped, their components are released. Additionally, onions are rich in flavonoid antioxidants, which are known to have anti-inflammatory properties and may help prevent cancer. Along with garlic and yellow onions, try leeks, chives, shallots, and scallions.

## 10. Tomatoes

Lycopene, vitamins C and E, beta-carotene, and flavonol antioxidants, to mention just a few, are just a few of the many components that tomatoes have that are good for your health. Particularly, lycopene guards against cardiovascular disease, UV-induced skin damage, and prostate cancer.

Cooking tomatoes increases lycopene absorption; one cup of tomato sauce has ten times as much lycopene as one cup of chopped, raw tomatoes. Also bear in mind that healthy fats, such as nuts or a nut-based dressing, help carotenoids, such as lycopene, be absorbed more effectively. As a result, enjoy your tomatoes in a salad with nuts or a nut-based dressing for an added nutritional boost. To avoid the endocrine disruptor BPA in can liners, another option is to purchase chopped and crushed tomatoes in glass jars rather than cans.